Guide Lines for the Preparation of Tables of Food Composition

D. A. T. Southgate

Guide Lines for the Preparation of Tables of Food Composition

With Contributions by
J.C. Somogyi, Rüschlikon-Zürich
E.M. Widdowson, Cambridge

11 tables

S. Karger · Basel · München · Paris · London · New York · Sydney 1974

S. Karger · Basel · München · Paris · London · New York · Sydney
Arnold-Böcklin-Strasse 25, CH–4011 Basel (Switzerland)

Printed in Switzerland by Thür Offsetdruck AG, Pratteln
ISBN 3–8055–1780–7

Contents

National Food Composition Tables

General Considerations and Introductory Remarks

J.C. Somogyi

President of the Group of European Nutritionists, Rüschlikon, Zurich

The importance of reliable food composition tables can be assumed as generally known. From the exactness of their data depends the correct results of many nutritional and dietetic investigations. They play, for instance, a great role in the evaluation of nutritional surveys, or in the planning and calculation of various diets – to mention only two of the more important examples.

On the other hand, we know that the given values of nutrient content for the same foodstuff also often differ in the various comprehensive tables. The reasons for this are manifold, e.g. the diversity of the material used and/or the analytical methods employed, the non-uniform expression and conception of food tables, as well as the carrying over of previously incorrect data from the older editions into the new tables, etc. But also the variation in the composition, and the difference in the nomenclature of the same food in several countries, play a role.

These were the main reasons why the Group of European Nutritionists decided in 1970 to form a Working Party, to discuss and work out the general principles which have to be considered in the preparation of national food composition tables. Further, it was planned to summarize the results of the meetings of this Working Party in a report.

The report, drawn up following the discussions of the Working Party, is presented in this booklet, entitled 'Guide Lines for the Preparation of National Food Composition Tables', the author of which is Dr. *D. Southgate,* Cambridge (UK). The members of the Working Party who all contributed valuable work for the successful completion of this publication are: Dr. *E.M. Widdowson* (Great Britain) Chairman; Mrs. *D.L. Bocobo* (FAO, Rome); Prof. *R. Buzina* (Yugoslavia); Prof. *C. den Hartog* (Netherlands); Prof. *F. Fidanza* (Italy) Co-Chairman; Prof. *O. Högl* (Switzerland); Dr. *K. Lindner* (Hungary); Prof. *J.C. Somogyi* (Switzerland); Dr. *D.A.T. Southgate* (Great Britain); Prof. *A. Szczygiel* (Poland); Prof.

O. Turpeinen (Finland); Dr. *S.I. Westin* (Sweden) and Prof. *W. Wirths* (Federal Republic of Germany).

In connection with such a monograph, several questions can be raised: What is the origin of such food composition tables? When were they first prepared? How have they developed in the course of the years?

An answer to the latter questions is given by the interesting contribution of Dr. *E.M. Widdowson,* in which is summarized extremely well, the evolution of food composition tables by the example of Great Britain. Her article 'A Brief History of British Food Composition Tables', included in this booklet, completes excellently the 'Guide Lines' by Dr. *Southgate.*

Further important questions are as follows: Are national food composition tables really necessary? Would it not be more economic and easier to have comprehensive tables prepared by international organizations like FAO? I think both are indispensable, and in addition, also comprehensive tables for some regions.

The main reasons for the necessity for national food tables can be considered, among others, that some foods are prepared and eaten in a certain country only, or the same name products are produced in various countries, but with different compositions.

For example – as far as I know – the meat speciality called 'Bindenfleisch' or 'Bündnerfleisch', prepared from beef by air drying, is made only in Switzerland. It is characterized by a very low fat content (6 %) and used, therefore, in diets for weight reduction. The composition of such a product can be contained only in a national food table. Similar is the situation for some local cheese sorts like the 'Stilton' in Great Britain or the 'riccotta' (a kind of cottage cheese) in Italy.

With great probability the first food composition table was published about 150 years ago. An indication of it was found in the 'Handbuch der Physiologie des Gesamtstoffwechsels und der Fortpflanzung, Erster Teil, Physiologie des allgemeinen Stoffwechsels und der Ernährung' by *C. von Voit* (1). He writes on page 417 the following: 'Auf Grund der in den Nahrungsmitteln enthaltenen festen Teile und extraktiven Materien entstand die erste Nutritionsskala von *Percy und Vaquelin* (2) in 1818.'

Their article entitled 'Sur la qualité nutritive des aliments comparés entre eux' naturally cannot be compared with food composition tables as they are used nowadays. It was, however, a first step in the direction to know more about the composition and nutritive value of various foods. *Percy and Vaquelin* carried out these investigations by order of the minister of the 'Département de l'Intérieur', who was interested to know, in connection with the food supply in prisons, how, and to what extent, certain food items, e.g. potatoes, could be replaced by other vegetables.

It seems to me of interest to publish a page of the 'nutrition scale' of *Percy and Vaquelin,* which is a true reproduction of the original (table I).

It took nearly a century till the first food composition tables, in the sense that we are familiar with today, were published in the United States (1896) (3) and in Germany (1878) (4).

Over the past 40–50 years, national food composition tables have been produced in several European countries. Only a few examples should be mentioned.

The evolution of such tables in *Great Britain* is summarized in the above-mentioned paper of Dr. *Widdowson.*

In *Germany* was not only prepared the first European food composition table by *König* in 1878 (4), but here appeared one of the most comprehensive tables of the present day entitled: 'Die Zusammensetzung der Lebensmittel-Nährwerttabellen' by *Souci, Fachmann and Kraut* in 1962 (5).

In *Finland,* there has been a long-standing interest in food composition. The first food tables were published as early as 1925. More extensive food composition tables were prepared in 1935 by the Central Organization of Agricultural Societies. This book contained values for composition of various foods based partly on their own laboratory analyses. In the latest edition, the values for vitamins and minerals have been taken over from the literature. These are, however, progressively replaced by direct analytical values.

In *Switzerland* and *Italy,* the first national food composition tables were produced in 1944 and in 1946, respectively. These were largely compiled from values given in the FAO-tables (6). The data of the composition of many food items, however, resulted from direct analyses.

While the food tables in the *Netherlands* were originally compiled from values in the literature, in the current edition over 80 % of the values are based on analyses made in various Dutch laboratories. The tables are generally revised every 2 years.

In other European countries, e.g. in *Hungary, Poland and Sweden,* the first national food composition tables were published between 1950–60, after a sufficient number of foods had been analysed to enable the preparation of food tables. Also in these countries analytical work continues and the food tables are constantly being revised and completed. In Hungary, for instance, since 1951 when the first food tables were published, seven revised editions have appeared, the latest being in 1972 (7).

Table I

Noms des Végétaux.	Eau sur 500 gra.	Matière desséchée sur 500 gra.	Matière extractive sur 500 gra.	Cendres et substance corticale.	*Observations.*
Pain de 4 livres ordinaire.	125	375	»	très-peu.	Donne un produit acide à la distillation.
Viande maigre de bœuf.	350	170	»	très-peu.	Donne un produit essentiellement alcalin à la distillation.
Pommes de terre.	375	125	8	»	Produit acide à la distillation.
Navets.	460	40	23	$\frac{1}{500}$	Donne un produit acide à la distillation.
Carottes.	428 ½	71 ½	36	1 ½	Produit acide à la distillation.
Choux	460 ½	39 ½	19,8	$\frac{1}{500}$	Produit alcalin à la distillation.
Épinards.	428	72	28 ½	$\frac{1}{100}$	Produit très-alcalin à la distillation.
Haricots secs.	»	500	»	substance corticale. 40	Produit alcalin à la distillation.
Féves sèches.	»	500	»	55	Produit ammoniacal à la distillation.
Pois secs.	»	500	»	35	*Idem.*
Riz.	»	»	»	»	Produit acide à la distillation.
Lentilles.	»	500	»	27,5	Produit alcalin à la distillation.

It is interesting to mention, that in the current edition of the Swedish (8) and the Hungarian food composition tables (7), the energy values of foods are expressed, not only in kcalories, but also in kjoules. As far as I know, these are the first books on food composition, in which both energy values are included. It is very probable, that in the future editions of other national food tables, the same arrangements will be made.

Finally, I would like to thank all those who assisted in the organization of the meetings of the Working Party and in the preparation of this volume. A special debt of gratitude is due to the Green Meadow Foundation for its support.

References

1 *Von Voit, C.:* Physiologie des allgemeinen Stoffwechsels und der Ernährung. Handbuch der Physiologie des Gesamtstoffwechsels und der Fortpflanzung, vol. 6 (Vogel, Leipzig 1881).

2 *Percy, P.F. et Vaquelin, N.L.:* Sur la qualité nutritive des aliments comparés entre eux. Bull. Fac. méd., Paris *6:* 75–91 (1818).

3 *Atwater, W.O. and Woods, C.D.:* The chemical composition of American food materials. US Off. Expt. Stas., Expt. Sta. Bul. 28 (1896).

4 *König, J.:* Chemie der menschlichen Nahrungs- und Genussmittel (Springer, Berlin 1878).

5 *Souci, S.W.; Fachmann, W. und Kraut, H.:* Die Zusammensetzung der Lebensmittel-Nährwerttabellen (Wissenschaftl. Verlagsgesellsch., Stuttgart 1962).

6 *Chatfield, C.:* Food composition tables. Minerals and vitamins for international use. FAO, Rome 1954.

7 *Tarján, R. és Lindner, K.:* Tápanyagtáblázat (Medicina Könyvkiadó, Budapest 1972).

8 *Abramson, E.:* Kosttabell (Läromedelsförlagen, Stockholm 1971).

Author's address: Prof. Dr. *J.C. Somogyi,* Institute for Nutritional Research, Seestrasse 72, *CH–8803 Rüschlikon-Zurich* (Switzerland)

Guide Lines for the Preparation of Tables of Food Composition

D.A.T. Southgate

Dunn Nutritional Laboratory, University of Cambridge and Medical Research Council, Cambridge

General Principles

An overriding principle in the preparation of food tables, whether for national, regional or international use, is the consideration of their purpose. This should include both the needs of the potential users of the tables and the various ways in which the values in the tables are likely to be employed. This is important because only rarely will it be possible to encompass the needs of all types of users and usage in a single publication.

The purpose of tables of food composition can be seen as falling into four categories: (i) The planning of prescribed diets; (ii) the calculation of the intake of nutrients by individuals or groups of people such as in food consumption surveys of population groups; (iii) the planning of food supplies for population groups or countries as a whole, and (iv) for teaching and research.

These guide lines envisage that at the national level at least two types of tables are desirable. The first would be comprehensive, the tables would cover all important foodstuffs and take account of the variations in composition found in nature and describe the causes of variability in composition, where they are known.

The second would be shorter, prepared basically for the nutritionist and physician, and would contain values for the nutrients in most foods commonly eaten in the country concerned. The coverage of nutrients would not be so extensive nor would measures of variation in composition be given. Although this version would be intended for a user with some professional nutritional training, the increasing interest of the general public in nutritional matters makes it desirable that some general nutritional information should be included in the text.

Tables for specialised users such as diabetics and teachers of elementary nutrition could be derived from these basic tables. It is not proposed here to consider tables for specialised users of this kind.

In these guide lines the two types of table will be designated *Comprehensive* and *National,* although the two categories are not mutually exclusive.

The Comprehensive tables visualised in these guide lines may appear to represent 'counsels of perfection', and it is recognised that national priorities may not permit the preparation of two types of table in a particular country. In fact the volume of work involved in the preparation of comprehensive tables is so extensive that in the first instance, these tables need only be prepared by a few countries or on a cooperative, multinational basis.

Value of National Tables

In general, tables based on analyses of the foods eaten in the country concerned are desirable. Where, however, there is a considerable international movement of a food commodity, values obtained from the analysis of the food in other countries would be acceptable. Seasonal variations in the proportions of home-produced to imported items consumed should, however, be taken into account.

For many foods and some nutrients there is considerable uniformity in composition, for example the amino-acid composition of lean meat, and in these cases the international values can be used with confidence.

Values given for cooked items should take differences in regional methods of preparation into account.

Revision Procedures

Changes in food technology, animal and plant husbandry, packaging and marketing methods make it desirable that the food composition tables be regularly and thoroughly revised. It is important that those concerned with nutrition should be aware of the effects of changing food technologies and this can only be achieved if there is some regular provision for revision.

Selection of Food Items

This depends to a great extent on the resources available for the preparation of the tables, but in general it should be as extensive as possible, particularly in the Comprehensive tables. In the initial stages of the preparation of the tables it is useful to compile a complete list of all the foods eaten in the country. From this list the order of priority for the collection of values can be assigned, if possible on the basis of food consumption statistics. If limitations of some kind restrict the number of items which can be included then the first priority should be given to the staple items of the diet and other items which are important sources of one or more essential nutrients in the national diet.

Values for the food both raw and when prepared for consumption should be given. The method of preparation should be described in detail in the Comprehensive tables and more briefly in the National tables. The composition of prepared foods will vary according to the method of preparation, particularly in the case of some more labile nutrients. Nevertheless, values for the composition of foods 'as consumed' are essential for many users, and if the method of preparation is described the values published will be useful as a guide to the changes to be anticipated on preparing the food by another method.

In the case of proprietary foods it may be necessary to restrict the items to stable, well-established ones, unless frequent revision of the tables is possible. It is probably undesirable to use proprietary names in the tables, unless these are essential to identify the foods in question. However, the compilers of food composition tables should aim at developing a good working relationship with the food manufacturing industry, and close consultation with the industry should form a normal part of the procedure in producing food composition tables.

Specification of Food Items

The description of the items in the tables should be as precise as possible to enable the unequivocal identification of a particular food and the part of that food to which the published values apply. Identification will often involve the listing of local synonyms in the index. In the case of plant foods and some animal foods, fish in particular, the scientific taxonomic (i.e. Latin) name should also be given, preferably in the table with the values for its composition or alternatively in an appendix.

The composition of commercial varieties of fruits and vegetables may be different and the varieties to which the values apply should be given in the Comprehensive tables; the average consumer of vegetables may have no knowledge of the actual variety purchased and in the National tables a footnote referring to textual comment on the variation in composition between different commercial varieties may be considered sufficient.

Where foods are covered by legislation with regard to labelling in a particular country, the description of these items should be made in the approved legal fashion, with the popular synonyms if appropriate.

Selection of Nutrients

The Comprehensive tables should contain values for as many nutrients as possible. The National tables on the other hand should give values for a more selected range of nutrients. Both tables should, however, give values for the proportions of waste in the foodstuff as purchased and any changes in weight during preparation for consumption.

The production of extensive tables of amino- or fatty-acid composition may be unnecessary for the majority of users of National food tables. These data should be available in the Comprehensive tables. Where, however, Comprehensive tables are not available for a particular country the coverage of nutrients in the National tables needs to be more extensive. This increased coverage should be made on a selective basis, depending on the requirements of the users of the National tables concerned and on the relative availability and applicability of Comprehensive tables prepared in another country.

Table I gives a list of the nutrients that seem desirable in Comprehensive tables together with the possible simplifications which could be considered in the less extensive National tables.

Many of the nutrients given in the table do not require definition or justification for their inclusion. However, it is necessary to define others more precisely. The list is not intended to be exclusive. Moreover, it is not necessary to give values for all the nutrients for all foodstuffs; indeed, a great measure of selectivity is desirable because of the time-consuming nature of, and expense involved in analytical work.

Water

This should be given in both types of table. The inclusion of values for water is important as it enables values for other nutrients in different tables for the same or similar foodstuffs to be compared on a similar moisture basis.

The use of a common moisture content as a basis of expressing the composition of particular foods, e.g. cereals, has some advantages, but this method and that of expression on a dry matter basis, are not convenient for the majority of users.

Table I. Constituents which are desirable in 'Comprehensive tables of food composition' together with possible simplifications for 'National tables'

Constituent	Possible simplification in 'National tables'[1]
Water	
Total nitrogen	
Protein (total-N minus non-protein derived-N) × factor	
Protein-N	Not necessary for most users
Amino-acid composition including 'available lysine'	The tables could be restricted to foods containing appreciable amounts of protein and the more important vegetables
Other nitrogenous substances, purines etc.	Probably not necessary
Fat, total	
Fat, glyceride	Not necessary
Fatty acid composition	The values could be restricted to the more important foods and the fatty acids grouped
Phospholipids	Not necessary
Sterols	Cholesterol values only
Available carbohydrate	
Individual sugars and available polysaccharides	

1 No entry in this column indicates that the coverage required is similar to that in the Comprehensive tables. It assumes that the information would be available for specialised users.

Table I (continued)

Constituent	Possible simplification in 'National tables'[1]
Unavailable carbohydrate	
Components of unavailable carbohydrate including lignin	Not necessary
Alcohol	
Organic acids	Only where they may contribute to the energy value of the food
Energy value	
Inorganic constituents: Na, K, Ca, Mg, P, Cl, Fe, Cu, Zn, Mn, Co, I, F	Of the trace elements only Fe may be necessary
Vitamin A activity	
Retinol	Probably not necessary for all foods but some indication is desirable where the major source of activity is due to carotenoids
Carotenoids	
Vitamin D	
Vitamin C	
Thiamin	
Riboflavin	
Niacin, total and available	Total values should be qualified with remarks about the occurrence of unavailable forms in cereals

1 No entry in this column indicates that the coverage required is similar to that in the Comprehensive tables. It assumes that the information would be available for specialised users.

Table I (continued)

Constituent	Possible simplification in 'National tables'[1]
Niacin equivalents of tryptophan present	
Folic acid, with separation of conjugates	Values given for only the monoglutamyl form of pteroylglutamic acid
Vitamin B_{12}	
Tocopherols, with separation of different forms	Values given for α-form only
Vitamin B_6, with separation of three forms	May not be necessary to give values for the different forms

1 No entry in this column indicates that the coverage required is similar to that in the Comprehensive tables. It assumes that the information would be available for specialised users.

Protein

This should be based on the total nitrogen minus the non-protein nitrogen multiplied by a factor related to the amino-acid composition of the food.

Protein-Nitrogen and Non-Protein Nitrogen

Some foods contain appreciable concentrations of non-protein nitrogen, in particular fish and other marine foods, and it is important to distinguish between protein and non-protein nitrogen in these foods. The same is true to a lesser extent for vegetables, where a proportion of the total nitrogen may be lost by leaching into the cooking water. Proprietary foods occasionally contain a large proportion of their total nitrogen as non-protein nitrogen, and where this is derived from amino acids and peptides these should be included in the calculation of protein. Where the non-protein nitrogen is derived from compounds not related to protein it should be excluded in the calculation of protein.

Fat, Glyceride

The inclusion of this item is desirable in Comprehensive tables, primarily for use in the calculation of the energy value of the food and also because of the interest in glycerides from animal and vegetable sources. The widespread and increasing use of mono- and diglycerides in the food manufacturing industries is an additional reason for its inclusion.

Phospholipids

The different classes of these substances should be given in comprehensive tables because of their wide usage as emulsifying agents, and their physiological properties.

Sterols

The most important sterol from the nutritional viewpoint was thought at one time to be cholesterol, but the other sterols, e.g. sitosterol, are of nutritional significance and these should be given in the comprehensive tables.

Available Carbohydrates

These include all the sugars known to be glucogenic in man and the polysaccharides hydrolysed by the endogenous secretions of the human digestive tract (52, 74).

Unavailable[1] *Carbohydrate*

These include the structural polysaccharides of the plant cell wall, pectic substances, cellulose and the hemicelluloses, lignin (not strictly a carbohydrate) and the non-starch reserve polysaccharides such as inulin (52, 53). These are, in general, not hydrolysed by endogenous secretions although they may be degraded in the gastro-intestinal tract by the microflora (52, 55, 77).

Organic Acids

These are only important in a limited number of foodstuffs and should be included on a selective basis. Values need only be given for fruits and fruit products (including beverages) and a few vegetables, particularly those preserved in acetic acid.

Allocation of Priorities

The priorities in the choice of nutrients or foods included in the National tables depend very much on the country concerned. Where, for example, the diet is known to contain rich sources of preformed vitamin A it may be considered unnecessary to allocate analytical resources to the study of carotenoids, although ideally all nutrients and foods should be covered.

Methods for Collecting Values

These may be considered under two headings, *indirect,* that is from the literature and unpublished sources, and *direct* by analysis under the control of the compilers of the tables.

Indirect, from Published and Unpublished Sources

This, although it is a less satisfactory method may, in some cases, be the only practicable way of preparing extensive tables. It is, however, not an easy exercise, because it requires critical assessment by someone experi-

1 Unavailable constituents of foods are defined as substances which are not utilised by the human organism either because they are not absorbed or, if absorbed, cannot be metabolised.

enced in food analysis, of the values available. In this matter it is desirable to draw upon the experience of specialist institutes within a country.

This assessment involves the nature of the sample analysed and whether it can be considered a 'normal' food, that is comparable with a similar food grown and prepared in essentially the same way as it would be in the country for which the tables are being prepared.

A considerable amount of the work described in the published literature on food composition is experimental in nature. For the purposes of the compiler of food tables only values obtained from 'control' groups can be used, but even here the compiler has to be sure that the methods of husbandry, either plant or animal, are typical of normal commercial practice. In the case of animals the compiler must satisfy himself that the animals were both reared and slaughtered in a similar way to that used for animals eaten in his own country.

The methods of analysis used by the authors must also be closely scrutinised and any departures from standard accepted procedures noted and assessed. This makes it incumbent on the authors of this type of publication to describe their methods fully.

The compiler must evaluate the various studies on the same foodstuff; in general greater weight will tend to be given to studies where a larger number of samples has been analysed.

The various stages of this assessment must be applied to both published and unpublished sources of values. In many cases it is difficult to decide whether differences reported by different authors for the amounts of a nutrient in the same food are genuine, that is due to natural variation, or are analytical or sampling artefacts. Careful specification of the samples analysed when reported in the literature would assist in this matter and table II gives the type of specific detail that the compiler of food tables needs.

The values for a nutrient given in the tables should be a representative one and this may not necessarily be the mean of all reported values; its choice depends, in the final analysis, on the critical judgement of the compilers after the completion of the assessment of all the available values. It therefore should be designated a *selected value* and the criteria used in its selection carefully described in the tables themselves.

Direct, by Analysis

This is the most satisfactory method. If the analytical work is not directly under the control of the compilers of the tables, frequent discus-

Table II. Specification of samples. Details of the description of samples ideally required by compilers of food composition tables

General heading	Details required
Name of food	Common name, with local synonyms. Scientific taxonomic name with variety where known
Origin of food	Plant foods Locality where grown, with details of soil conditions and fertiliser treatments.
	Animals products Locality and method of husbandry and slaughter (where applicable)
Nature of sample collected	Place and time of collection. Number of samples collected. Whether purchased retail. State in which it was purchased, e.g. raw, prepared, deep frozen, pre-packed, etc.
Treatment of samples before analysis	Conditions and length of storage. Preparative treatment, including details of material discarded as waste. Method of cooking (where applicable)
Analysis	Details of material analysed. Analytical methods used, with appropriate references and details of any modifications used
Method of expression of results[1]	Statistical treatment of analytical values. Whether expressed on a 'as purchased', 'edible matter' or 'dry matter', etc. basis

1 Whenever results are expressed on a basis *other* than fresh weight, details should be given so that the results can be calculated back to this basis.

sion and consultation with the analysts concerned is essential and it is in this particular area that experience of food analysis is a valuable qualification for the compiler of tables.

The analysis of foods for nutritional purposes is often outside the field of primary training of many analytical chemists and the discussions recommended are essential in maintaining the nutritional bias of food composition tables, and are usually of mutual benefit to both nutritionist and analyst.

If values are to be obtained by analysis for inclusion in the tables, provided that the various analytical criteria discussed later are met, the only limiting feature in the reliability of the values obtained is the collection and treatment before analysis of the samples of foods. This is discussed in the following section.

Sampling

The importance of analysing *representative samples* cannot be overemphasised, particularly so because the majority of the users of food composition tables, especially tables of the National type, will use the single value (be it mean or selected) given in the tables and will not usually be in a position to use statistical estimates of variations in composition. Therefore the values given in the tables must be based on samples which are representative of the average composition of the particular foodstuffs.

Selection of the Sample

In deciding on the way in which the representative sample should be made up, use should be made of a number of different types of information which bear on the factors which influence the average composition of the foodstuff.

National food consumption statistics can often be used to ensure that the samples reflect trends in the seasonal and regional pattern of consumption of the food. This should also take into account the proportions of home-grown or produced foods and imported items eaten at different times of the year.

Statistical data of an economic nature, either collected by a government or the retail trade concerned, can also be used to ensure that the samples are collected in the correct proportions from different types of retail outlets where the food is purchased (21). In this connection it is important that the proportions purchased for domestic and institutional use be correctly reflected in the sample, especially because foods purchased for hospitals, schools and canteens will be amongst the latter.

In the final selection of the samples, where for example there are wide variations in price and/or quality, the average price for a particular foodstuff derived from governmental or trade sources is often a good guide to the 'average' sample. The representative sample of the food which will be used to provide the values for the tables, will therefore be made up from a number of subsamples, the selection of which will be determined by the procedure described above.

Sampling Protocol

The definition of the representative sample in the manner described above determines the type of sampling protocol required for a particular food or group of foods.

Foods which show seasonal variations in composition should be sampled throughout the year, and those that show variations from region to region should be sampled in the different regions. This means that for some foods an elaborate sampling protocol will be necessary, involving the purchasing of subsamples in different regions and throughout the year. Other foods which show less variation in composition can be sampled according to a much simpler procedure. The number of subsamples will be determined by the type of food; in general a food which is quantitatively important in the diet would warrant a larger number of subsamples than a food consumed in smaller quantities. As a general rule a minimum of ten subsamples is suggested.

To some extent sampling is an art which can be acquired by practice, and the sampler must be prepared to adapt his procedure for each particular food, bearing in mind the nature of the food and its associated technology (if any).

For some foods, recognised procedures for sampling have been adopted and used for many years (2) and these should be taken into account when these foods are being sampled.

Size of the Subsample

This will depend on the type of food, the number of analyses contemplated, and on whether the subsamples are to be pooled before analysis or analysed separately.

Treatment of the Subsamples

Once the food has been collected the subsamples must be treated from the time of collection in such a way as to avoid losses of nutrients or contamination from external sources.

In general, deep-freezing (−20 °C) in a sealed container is a useful method of preservation, but care must be taken to ensure that losses of moisture do not occur. The activity of the more labile vitamins, especially retinol, vitamin C and the tocopherols will, however, be lost under these conditions and immediate pretreatment of a portion of the subsample is essential. The details are discussed under the methods of analysis for these vitamins.

Analysis of the Representative Sample

If information on natural and other variations in the composition of a food are required then the individual subsamples must be analysed separately. This involves a large amount of time-consuming and therefore, expensive, analytical work and is probably only justifiable for foods which form a major part of the diet or where there are suspected seasonal or regional variations in composition. This may be the case for some fruits and vegetables, particularly where vitamin C is concerned.

The values obtained on the separate subsamples are then combined proportionately, according to the information used in deciding the make-up of the representative sample, to provide the values for the tables themselves.

Alternatively the individual subsamples are pooled in the correct proportions to provide a large sample representative of the food in question, which is then analysed to provide the values for the tables. This is probably the most acceptable procedure (53), especially from the viewpoint of the allocation of analytical resources. The pooling of the subsamples must be carried out with care, and the thorough mixing of them may pose technical problems, particularly if it is necessary to avoid contact with metals because trace metal analyses are to be performed.

The representative sample produced by pooling the separate subsamples may be too large to be handled conveniently in the laboratory. Its size should be reduced by the conventional 'quartering' method or by serial division of the well-mixed sample into aliquot parts.

Apart from the loss of information on variations in composition of a food the procedure of pooling subsamples to provide a representative sample for analysis gives values which are adequate, provided that the representative sample has been collected with care.

Modes of Expression

It is difficult to separate the discussion of the mode of expression chosen for a nutrient from the methods used in its measurement. This section is therefore mainly concerned with setting out some general principles.

National preferences exist for the method of expressing nutrients (and for methods of analysis) and in the case of many nutrients the choice of the best method of expression is not clear-cut.

Whenever possible the nomenclature and mode of expression should follow the recommendations of the various expert committees set-up by the international agencies (30, 31, 42). Occasionally, the mode of expression of a nutrient chosen by a particular country may differ from these international recommendations and, since the dietitians and physicians may have to use their national tables in conjunction with their own countries' recommended dietary allowances or intakes (26, 30, 31), it is essential to retain some flexibility of outlook.

It is important to stress that the compilers of food composition tables must define clearly the terminology and modes of expression they have chosen to use.

Statistical Expression of Variations in Composition

In both types of table the number of samples analysed should be given and in the Comprehensive tables, in addition to the mean value for a constituent, some appropriate statistical parameter to describe the observed variation, such as the standard deviation or the standard error of the mean. Where the number of samples analysed is small the use of the standard deviation is not recommended and it should also not be used where the values for the composition of the food show a grossly skewed distribution.

Where sufficient numbers of analytical values are available a percentile system is useful to give a measure of the variation observed.

The majority of users of National tables will not be in a position to use statistical information. In these tables textual and footnote guidance on variation is probably all that is necessary.

Bases for Expression

Wherever possible, constituents should be expressed on a weight per weight of food basis except in the case of the amino-acids and fatty acids, where weight of amino acid per g N and per 100 g of total fatty acids are the preferable methods of expression, respectively. When vitamins are expressed in terms of equivalents (30, 31) it is important that the precise method of calculation is described in the text. In comprehensive tables the basic analytical values used in the calculation of vitamin activities in terms of equivalents should be given.

The preferred mode of expression for the individual vitamins will be discussed in the analytical section which follows.

According to the conventions of the Systeme International the weight of food used as the base should be the kilogram (65). This convention has some advantage in that the values expressed as mg/kg are equivalent to parts per million (p.p.m.). This is used extensively in food technology and is useful for food composition values on an 'as purchased' basis. The 100 g basis is, however, more familiar to the majority of users of National food tables and 100 g is closer to the normal sizes of portions of foods eaten. Probably the ideal would be to express 'as purchased' values per kg and 'as eaten' values per 100 g.

Methods of Analysis

As the primary object of tables of food composition is *nutritional* the most appropriate method for the determination of a nutrient is that which reflects the nutritive value of the foodstuff for man. This method may not be the best with regard to analytical characteristics such as reproducibility, precision or speed of analysis, and the nutritional analysis of foods requires a different approach from that required for food analysis for legislative purposes or quality control.

Before reviewing the analytical methods for the various constituents there are some general points which apply in all cases.

First, it is the responsibility of the person in charge of the analytical work to ensure, by means of the examination of known mixtures and by recovery tests, that the procedures adopted give satisfactory results.

Second, where different analysts are involved, either within the same laboratory or in independent laboratories, samples should be exchanged for comparative analysis.

Third, the procedures adopted should be given by reference in the comprehensive tables, together with a description of any unpublished modification used.

Fourth, the selection of the most appropriate method for any particular nutrient in any given food should be accompanied by a description of the appropriate analytical precautions (2, 28).

Review of Analytical Methods and their Limitations

In this review of analytical methods an attempt has been made to suggest suitable methods. However, in many cases the choice of the most appropriate method is not clear-cut and it is not intended that these guide lines should lay down methodology in an inflexible fashion. Furthermore, in some cases the preferred method may require extensive instrumentation and here alternative procedures, often of comparable accuracy but more time-consuming, have been suggested.

The selection of references to the methods proved extremely difficult because of the many alternative modifications described in the literature, and the approach adopted has been to select the generally preferred principle of analysis and to quote, where possible a review, or some exemplary references.

Water

Three procedures are given in table III; of these, freeze-drying is probably the best as it allows the use of large samples and because the moisture is removed under mild conditions, so that many other nutrients

Table III. Water

Available methods	Comments on limitations
Freeze-drying	Mild and efficient if followed by removal of residual moisture *in vacuo* over P_2O_5
Vacuum oven at 60 °C	Most rapid if a slow leak of dry air is passed through the oven
Air oven at 100–105 °C	To minimise destruction of sugars and fats the time at high temperature should be kept as short as possible

may be measured subsequently in the freeze-dried material. The method itself also produces a sample which is in many cases readily homogenised. Some residual moisture remains after freeze-drying and this must be removed under reduced pressure over a suitable desiccant. The disadvantage of this procedure is the cost of equipment.

Drying in a vacuum oven (2) is preferable to drying in an air-oven at a higher temperature. Drying in an air oven at 100 ∿ 105 °C is, however, a widely used procedure and, while it is undesirable to subject many foods to this type of procedure, for most nutritional purposes the methods which do not result in the obvious destruction of a constituent such as the caramelisation of sugars or oxidation of fats are applicable and will give similar, if not identical results.

Where a food contains alcohol this will be lost during drying and the alcohol must be measured separately and deducted from the apparent water content.

Nitrogen and Nitrogenous Constituents

The various analytical methods are summarised in table IV.

Total Nitrogen

This is usually measured by one of the many variants of the Kjeldahl method. The choice of catalyst and digestion conditions have been reviewed by *Fleck and Munro* (33), who recommend the use of mercury-based mixtures, although for most nutritional work the choice of catalyst is not critical. The temperature achieved during digestion, however, is and should be, between 370° and 410 °C.

The automatic determination of nitrogen, where the samples are digested automatically and the ammonia formed measured colorimetrically (71) is useful where large numbers of analyses have to be made and the instrumentation is available; although the accuracy of the results obtained by this method is not comparable to that obtained by the Kjeldahl method.

Protein-Nitrogen

This is most conveniently measured after precipitation of the protein and removal of the non-protein nitrogen. A large number of different precipitants have been used; all of them are to some extent empirical and need to be tested with the type of food under examination (84).

Table IV. Methods for nitrogen and nitrogenous constituents

Constituent	Available methods	Limiting factors	References
Total nitrogen	*Kjeldahl* procedure	'Catalyst' and conditions of digestion	(33)
	Automatic digestion and colorimetric measurement of ammonia formed	Cost of instrumentation	(71)
Protein	(Total nitrogen minus nitrogen from non-protein related substances) × factor	Factor should be specific for the food in question	(45, 99)
Protein-nitrogen	Measurement of total nitrogen after precipitation of protein and removal of non-protein nitrogen	Choice of precipitant	(84)
Amino-acid composition	Ion-exchange chromatography after acid hydrolysis with S-containing acids oxidised with performic acid before hydrolysis. Tryptophan measured after alkaline hydrolysis	Hydrolytic conditions are critical especially in the presence of carbohydrates	(63, 78) (69, 93) (58)
	Gas-liquid chromatography	Preparation of volatile derivatives	(37)
Available lysine	After reaction with fluoro-dinitro benzene	Interference from other constituents	(12, 15)
Other nitrogenous constituents	Specific biochemical procedures		(23, 60) (62)

Protein

For the purposes of food tables the application of a factor to the total nitrogen minus the nitrogen of non-protein derivation, or to the protein nitrogen determined directly, is adequate. The factor used for each particular food should be related to the percentage nitrogen in the proteins in the food and can be computed from the amino acid composition of the food. The indiscriminate use of N × 6.25 for protein is not desirable and some of the more appropriate factors are given in table V.

Amino-Acid Composition

Both the suggested methods require automatic instrumentation, and at the present time, procedures based on ion-exchange chromatography are the most widely used (63, 78). The limiting factor in these procedures is the hydrolytic stage, particularly in the presence of carbohydrate (69, 93). A high ratio of hydrolysing acid to sample is desirable and the hydrolysis is best performed in sealed tubes, either after evacuation or flushing with oxygen-free nitrogen (93).

It is essential to oxidise the sulphur-containing amino-acids, usually with performic acid (58), before hydrolysis.

Tryptophan may be measured after alkaline hydrolysis by ion-exchange chromatography or directly by a colorimetric procedure (38, 80).

The application of gas-liquid chromatographic techniques in the determination of amino-acids is limited at present by the preparation of suitable volatile derivatives (37). However, once these technical problems have been resolved the rapidity of procedures based on this principle would make them extremely attractive.

Available Lysine

The measurement of available lysine (15) should form part of the assessment of the amino-acid composition of a food. The main limitations seem to be the interference from other constituents, which can be eliminated by ion-exchange separation techniques (12). It is important that values for the food in both the raw and ready-to-consume forms are given.

Other Nitrogenous Constituents

Foods, especially fish and other marine foods, contain a wide range of nitrogenous substances and many foods contain appreciable amounts of nucleic acids. While many of these nitrogenous substances react with ninhydrin and can be separated by ion-exchange chromatography, the

Table V. Factors for the conversion of nitrogen values to protein[1] (g per g N). (Where no specific factor is given, 6.25 should be used on an interim basis until a more appropriate factor has been determined)

Animal products		Plant products	
foodstuff	factor	foodstuff	factor
Meat and fish	6.25	Wheat	
		whole	5.83
Gelatin	5.55	bran	6.31
		embryo	5.80
Milk and milk products	6.38	endosperm	5.70
Casein	6.40	Rice and rice flour	5.95
Human milk	6.37	Rye and rye flour	5.83
Eggs		Barley and barley flour	5.83
whole	6.25		
albumin	6.32	Oats	5.83
vitellin	6.12		
		Millet	6.31
		Beans	6.25
		Soya	5.71
		Nuts	
		almond	5.18
		brazil	5.46
		groundnut	5.46
		others	5.30

1 Based on values quoted in the literature (45, 99) and on calculations made by Dr. *K. Lindner.*

complex mixtures present in the 'non-protein-nitrogen' fraction make identification difficult, and for most substances specific biochemical procedures are often easier to apply. *Dawson et al.* (23) is a useful source of reference to methods for the isolation and estimation of the nitrogenous constituents found in foods, and methods for the measurement of nucleic acids have recently been reviewed (60).

Lipid Constituents

The methods for the various lipid constituents are summarised in table VI.

Fat, Total

In general, procedures based on continuous extraction of the dried food with a lipid solvent are not recommended and are given in the table solely because of their widespread use. They are known to give incomplete extraction from many foods (2, 5, 76) and also subject the extracted lipid to prolonged periods at high temperatures.

Procedures based on extraction with mixed solvents of the *Folch* type (35, 79) are to be preferred (5, 76), although the fats in some foods, e.g. eggs which contain high concentrations of phospholipids, may not be completely extracted without previous mild acid treatment.

The methods based on acid hydrolysis of the food followed by extraction with mixed solvents (2, 77) give complete extraction of lipid but tend to be time-consuming and they do not yield the lipid in state where it can be used for other qualitative work, unless appropriate precautions are taken to prevent oxidation by carrying out the extraction under nitrogen.

Fat, Glyceride

This can be estimated by difference after measuring the unsaponifiable matter present (2) or by calculation from the fatty acid composition of the sample. The proportions of tri-, di- and monoglycerides can be most conveniently measured after separation by thin-layer chromatography (81).

Fatty Acid Composition

Separation and measurement of the methyl esters by gas-liquid chromatography is unquestionably the method of choice, having entirely

Table VI. Methods for lipid constituents

Constituent	Available methods	Limiting factors	References
Fat, total	Mixed solvent (*Folch* type)	Rapid and complete under mild conditions	(5, 35) (76)
	Acid-hydrolysis followed by mixed solvent extraction	Complete extraction but under vigorous condition, time-consuming	(2, 77)
	Continuous extraction (*Soxhlet* type)	Incomplete extraction from many foods, time-consuming	(2, 19)
Fat, glyceride	By difference after measuring unsaponifiable fraction		(2, 19)
	By calculation from fatty acid content	Presence of phospholipids or cholesterol esters	(81)
Fatty-acid composition	Gas liquid chromatography of methyl esters	Obtaining quantitative methylation	(68, 83) (88)
Phospholipids	Total by measuring lipid-soluble phosphorus; specific biochemical methods		(1, 23)
Sterols	Gas liquid chromatography		(23, 51) (101)
	Specific colorimetric procedures	Specificity of methods	

superseded the older methods based on fractional crystallisation and distillation. The only limit to the accuracy of this method is the quantitative preparation of the methyl esters, which may be by interesterification (83) or reaction with diazomethane (68). The methods of preparation of the methyl esters have been recently reviewed (19, 83), and a simple procedure has been developed for serial analyses (88).

Phospholipids

Measurement of the lipid-solvent soluble phosphorus gives a useful measure of the total amounts of phospholipid present, but in general, specific biochemical procedures for the individual substances are to be preferred (1, 23).

Carbohydrates

The continued use of carbohydrate *by difference* in tables of food composition is not recommended and should be replaced by values based on direct analysis. The separation of the carbohydrates into two categories: *available,* that is carbohydrates which are digested and absorbed by the secretions of the human digestive tract and which are glucogenic in man, and unavailable, those which are not digested by man (52), which include the structural carbohydrates of the plant cell wall and lignin, remains a useful concept (36, 77). The methods are summarised in table VII.

Available Carbohydrate

Most procedures involve the separation of the free sugars from the polysaccharides by extraction with aqueous alcohol followed by their measurement either colorimetrically (36, 74) or enzymatically (8, 92). Starches and dextrins can be measured after hydrolysis either enzymatically (36, 54, 74) or after dilute acid hydrolysis using a glucose-specific enzymatic method. In some foods, particularly cereals, extraction with perchloric acid followed by colorimetric measurement gives reliable results (17).

Mode of Expression

It is suggested, to avoid confusion, that available carbohydrate be expressed as monosaccharides. Where a value is given as a disaccharide it should be multiplied by 1.05 and as starch by 1.1.

Table VII. Methods for carbohydrates, alcohol and organic acids

Constituent	Available methods	Limiting factors	References
Available carbohydrate	Extraction of free sugars and measurement by colorimetric procedures	Specificity of chemical procedures	(36, 74)
	Hydrolysis of starch enzymatically, measurement of glucose colorimetrically or enzymatically	Specificity of enzyme preparation used	(8, 54)
	Extraction of starch with perchloric acid followed by colorimetric measurement	Interference from other constituents	(17)
Constituent sugars	Ion-exchange chromatography	Cost of instrumentation	(34, 46, 47)
	Specific enzymatic procedures	Purity of enzyme preparations	(8, 92)
	Gas-liquid chromatography	Preparation of volatile derivatives	(9, 86)
Unavailable carbohydrates and the other components of the cell wall	Fractional extraction and hydrolysis	All procedures at present are empirical to a greater or lesser extent	(75, 95)
	Modifications of the classical fibre procedure based on 'normal-acid fibre'	Procedures for fibre were developed for work with the ruminant and underestimate the carbohydrates not digested by man	(95, 96)
Alcohol	Gas-liquid chromatography		
	Specific enzyme procedures		(8)
	Distillation		

Table VII (continued)

Constituent	Available methods	Limiting factors	References
Organic acids	Specific enzyme methods		
	Ion-exchange chromatography		(2, 8, 23)
	Thin-layer chromatography		(81)

Constituent Sugars

The individual sugars may be measured either using specific enzymatic assay techniques (8, 92) or colorimetrically after separation by ion-exchange chromatography (34, 46, 47). This latter procedure requires automatic instrumentation, but is to be preferred where a large number of different carbohydrate species are present, as in some fruits. Gas-liquid chromatography offers great potential use in this field (9, 86).

Unavailable Carbohydrates

These include the structural polysaccharides of the plant cell wall, pectins, cellulose and hemicelluloses, lignin (not strictly a carbohydrate) and the non-starch reserve polysaccharides such as inulin and the algal polysaccharides. This is an area where there are considerable gaps in our knowledge, both with regard to the analytical chemistry of these substances and their physiological properties in the gastro-intestinal tract.

In general, the classical method for 'crude fibre' is considered unsatisfactory because of its empirical nature and the variable composition of the fraction from food to food (2, 39).

Although analytical procedures are still to a large extent empirical, the measurement of lignin and cellulose should be made by one of the more recently developed procedures (75, 95, 96). Procedures developed for work in connection with the nutrition of the ruminant are not wholly satisfactory for human studies, where more research is required.

Alcohol

The use of gas-liquid chromatography or alternatively enzymatic procedures based on the use of alcohol dehydrogenase (8) seem preferable and more specific than the classical distillation methods, where the presence of other volatile substances interferes in the measurement of ethanol.

Organic Acids

These need only be measured in fruits and fruit products (including wines) and a few vegetables. Acetic acid, used as a preservative in many foods, should also be measured.

Of the available methods, assay with specific enzyme techniques (2, 8) appear to be preferable, although separation by ion-exchange chromatography or thin-layer chromatography followed by a colorimetric procedure gives satisfactory results with many foods (23, 81).

Inorganic Constituents

The methods for inorganic constituents are summarised in table VIII. In most cases, instrumental methods of analysis are considered preferably to the classical gravimetric or volumetric procedures, and in general offer greater specificity and sensitivity than many colorimetric methods. These older methods are still of value as reference procedures.

Whenever instrumental procedures are used, however, it is essential to ensure that interference from other constituents has been eliminated or controlled. This may be done either by the use of standard solutions containing the interfering substances in similar concentrations to those found in the samples being examined, or by the addition of substances which suppress the interference. This latter procedure is often of value in atomic absorption spectrophotometry.

Preparation of the Sample

For many elements the first stage in the analysis is the destruction of the organic matter in the food, which can be done either by ignition in a muffle furnace in a silica or platinum crucible, or by oxidation with hot concentrated acids, usually with mixtures of sulphuric, nitric or perchloric acids (51).

Some elements react with the material of the crucible (2, 67) or are converted into insoluble compounds during either dry-ashing or wet (acid) oxidation, and the possibility of this occurring in particular foods must be borne in mind by the analyst.

Table VIII. Methods for inorganic constituents

Constituent	Available methods	Limiting factors	References
Preparation of sample	Dry-ashing in a silica or platinum crucible	Temperature of ignition must be kept below 475 °C to avoid losses of Na and K. Some elements interact with the crucible	(2, 53, 67)
	Oxidation with concentrated acid i.e. wet-ashing	Formation of insoluble compounds	
Sodium potassium	Flame photometry, or atomic absorption spectrophotometry	Interference from other constituents must be controlled	(2, 51)
Calcium	(a) Atomic absorption spectrophotometry (b) Flame photometry	Interference effects in (a) and (b) must be controlled by addition of suitable reagents	(2)
	(c) Precipitation as the oxalate		
	(d) Compleximetric titration	(d) Requires careful control of the titration	
Magnesium Iron Copper Zinc Manganese Molybdenum Chromium Vanadium Selenium	Atomic absorption spectrophotometry	Interference effects need careful control	(67)
	Specific colorimetric procedures	Specificity of methods; usually time-consuming	
	Emmission spectrography	Very sensitive and rapid but often associated with low precision	(2)
Phosphorus	Colorimetrically	All phosphorus must be in the orthophosphate form	(32)

Table VIII (continued)

Constituent	Available methods	Limiting factors	References
Iodine	Microdistillation and titration		(13)
Fluorine	Microdistillation then colorimetrically		(13, 56, 70)
Chloride	Potentiometric titration		(22)

If the alkali metals are to be determined it is important to ensure that the temperature in the muffle furnace does not exceed 475 °C, as at higher temperatures, losses of these elements may occur by volatilisation (53).

The ash resulting from the dry-ashing is conveniently dissolved in hydrochloric acid and measurements made on the ash extract (53). The concentrated acid digestion mixture from the wet ashing procedure is diluted before analysis.

Sodium and Potassium

Either flame photometry or atomic absorption spectrophotometry provide the preferred methods. In both cases some mutual interference effects occur which are significant when one element is present in a great excess; this can usually be controlled by the use of appropriate standard solutions. In some cases phosphorus interferes in flame photometric measurements.

Calcium

Both flame photometry and atomic absorption spectrophotometry offer similar sensitivities. Phosphorus interferes in both procedures but the interference can usually be suppressed by the addition of lanthanum salts to the samples and standard solutions (2).

The classical method involving precipitation as the oxalate provides a useful reference procedure, but may give low results when the amounts of calcium to be measured are very small.

Compleximetric titration with a suitable chelating agent is satisfactory provided that the end-point of the titration is followed photometrically (2).

Magnesium

Atomic absorption spectrophotometry is the method of choice as it offers considerably greater specificity and sensitivity than any other procedure apart from activation analysis. Flame photometry can also be used if the appropriate precautions are taken in the preparation of the standard curves (51).

Phosphorus

Colorimetric measurement after conversion to the orthophosphate (32) is the preferred method. Either dry-ashing or wet (acid) digestion methods are applicable provided that any pyrophosphates formed during the destruction of the organic matter have been hydrolysed.

Chloride

In general either extraction with dilute nitric acid or oxidation with concentrated nitric acid in the presence of excess silver nitrate, followed by potentiometric titration (which is preferable to the classical Volhard titration) provide the preferred methods (22).

If a dry-ashing procedure is used it is necessary to ensure that the sample remains alkaline during the ashing (2).

Trace Elements

Any work with these elements requires scrupulous attention to laboratory technique with regard to the prevention of extraneous contamination if results of value are to be obtained.

The concentration of many of these constituents, particularly in plant products, is greatly affected by the soil in which they were grown and the fertiliser treatment they have received. It is essential, therefore, that the specification of the sample with regard to these characteristics is as complete as possible, if the results are to be of any significance.

Once the sample has been collected (or prepared ready for consumption) contact with metal of any kind must be scrupulously avoided. In this connection the presence of iron in the dust of most laboratories is an ever present source of contamination.

For most trace elements atomic absorption spectrophotometry provides the method of choice, although colorimetric procedures are available which are of variable specificity (67). The interference from other constituents in the food must be checked by the analyst.

Emission spectrography (2) provides a rapid and extremely sensitive procedure, and a large number of elements can be measured simultaneously. In general the precision of the method is not high, but its rapidity enables a large number of replicate measurements to be made on the same sample so that statistical analyses of the values obtained can be made to estimate the concentration in the sample.

Fluoride and Iodide

These require special microdistillation techniques (70); *Bowen* (13) describes these in detail in connection with procedures for activation analysis and the microdistillation procedure for fluoride can be followed by colorimetric measurement (56).

Vitamins

The methods for the vitamins are summarised in table IX together with the suggested mode of expression which should be used in tables of food composition.

In the determination of many vitamins the preliminary treatment of the sample is critical, in some cases to preserve the vitamin activity in the food when sampled and in others, particularly those of the B-complex, to ensure complete extraction (3, 40, 85).

Microbiological methods are frequently more specific than chemical ones (3, 82) for many vitamins, and in these cases the organism suggested is given a type culture number according to the American and British collections. The preparation of the culture media is often critical and the general principles have been reviewed in several papers (6, 7, 18, 40, 50, 72, 85).

Retinol

Rapid treatment of the sample with ethanolic potassium hydroxide is necessary to preserve the retinol activity, and after this the sample may be stored in the frozen state with little loss of activity. The saponification stage is critical and should be carried out under oxygen-free nitrogen with the period of saponification kept as short as possible (3, 40, 85) in order to minimise isomerisation. The analyst should confirm that the time of saponification used is appropriate for the food under examination.

Chromatographic separation followed by either spectrophotometric (14, 97) or colorimetric determination (16, 43, 73, 97) is the suggested method of analysis.

Table IX. Vitamins – methods and mode of expression

Constituent	Available methods	Mode of expression where different from a simple weight basis	References
Retinol	Saponification then either colorimetrically or spectrophotometrically after chromatographic separation	As retinol equivalents for Vitamin A activity: 1 μg retinol = 1 μg equivalent; 6 μg β-carotene = 1 μg equivalent; 12 μg of other active carotenoids	(14, 16, 43, 73, 82, 97)
Carotenoids			(10, 11, 87)
Vitamin D	Biological assay gas-liquid chromatography	Proposal for the use of cholecalciferol equivalent = 1 μg cholecalciferol or ergocalciferol ≡ 40 i.u. (for man)	(48, 61, 101)
Vitamin C	Fluorimetric assay		(2, 3, 27, 66, 81, 98)
	Preparation of dinitro phenyl hydrazones followed by thin-layer chromatography and colorimetric measurement. Titration with dichlorophenol-indophenol		
Thiamin[1]	Microbiologically with *L. viridescens* or *L. fermenti*		(2, 3, 25)
	Thiochrome method		(44)

1 Either acid or enzymatic treatment of the sample is essential to ensure complete liberation of the vitamins.

Table IX (continued)

Constituent	Available methods	Mode of expression where different from a simple weight basis	References
Riboflavin[1]	Microbiologically with *L. casei* or *Streptococcus zymogenes*		(2, 3)
	Fluorimetrically		(49)
Niacin[2] (total)	Colorimetrically	Expressed as niacin equivalents 1 mg equivalents = 1 mg niacin or niacinamide	(2, 6)
	Microbiologically with *L. plantarum*		(18)
(Available)	No accepted procedure, but bound forms can be separated by gel filtration		
Folic acid	Microbiologically with *L. casei* in presence and absence of conjugase with ascorbate as an antioxidant	Proposal to use folic acid equivalents ≡ 1 mg 'free folate' without conjugase treatment in view of the uncertainty about the availability of the higher conjugates	(20, 72) (91)
Vitamin B_{12}	Microbiologically with *L. leichmannii* after conversion to cyano form		(2, 90)

1 Either acid or enzymatic treatment of the sample is essential to ensure complete liberation of the vitamin.
2 Acid treatment of the sample is essential to ensure complete liberation of the vitamin.

Table IX (continued)

Constituent	Available methods	Mode of expression where different from a simple weight basis	References
Tocopherols	Separation by chromatography then measurement by colorimetric analysis	Proposal for α-tocopherol equivalent ≡ 1 mg α-tocopherol and at present to discount β-, γ- and δ-forms because of lower activity	(24, 29, 81, 94)
Vitamin B_6	Microbiologically with *Saccharomyces carlsbergensis*		(3, 4, 41)

Carotenoids

Spectrophotometric measurement after chromatographic separation is the suggested procedure (10, 11), although high pressure gas-liquid chromatography (87) allows the separation of the many isomeric forms.

Mode of Expression of Vitamin A Activity

The recommendation of the FAO/WHO expert committee (30) is that activity should be expressed in terms of retinol. The values to be assigned to the carotenoid pro-vitamins are summarised in the table. The recommendations of the United Kingdom (26) that the carotenoids in milk and milk products should be assigned a higher retinol equivalent value (2 μg carotenoids ≡ 1 μg retinol equivalents) is also recommended.

It is, however, important that whenever values are given as retinol equivalents, the method of calculation is given in the tables, and the basic analytical values should be given in the comprehensive tables.

Vitamin D

Biological assay procedures remain the accepted standard procedure (48) although it is envisaged that these will be replaced by procedures based on chromatographic separation and gas-liquid chromatography (61, 101).

The development of competitive protein-binding assay techniques for related substances in serum offers possibilities for the measurement of low concentrations of vitamin D and its metabolites in biological materials.

Mode of Expression

The use of a weight basis of expression is preferred, based on cholecalciferol, and related substances with different biological activities should be expressed on a cholecalciferol equivalent basis (26, 31).

Vitamin C

The terminology of the IUNS (42) should be used rather than ascorbic acid because of the biological activity of dehydroascorbic acid. Rapid extraction of the sample with metaphosphoric acid is essential (23).

The use of methods based on titration of dichlorophenol indophenol is not in general recommended; however, provided that appropriate precautions are taken (2, 3) the values obtained by this method are reliable for many foodstuffs. Procedures based on thin-layer chromatography separation of the 2:4 dinitrophenylhydrazones (66) following the procedure of *Vuilleumier* (98) or the fluorimetric procedure adopted by the AOAC (2) are preferred.

Thiamin

Preliminary digestion of the sample before extraction is essential (2, 3, 40, 82, 85, 89). Either microbiological assay using *Lactobacillus viridescens* (ATCC 12706) or *L. fermenti* (ATCC 9338) or the thiochrome method are suggested (2, 25, 44), provided that the sensitivity of the fluorimeter used is adequate (3).

Riboflavin

Most foodstuffs require preliminary treatment to hydrolyse carbohydrates which interfere with the extraction of riboflavin (2, 3, 40, 82, 85).

Fluorimetric measurement (49) or microbiological assay with *L. casei* ≡ *L. helveticus* (ATCC 7469) (2) or *Streptococcus zymogenes* (ATCC 10100 NCIB 7432) are suggested methods of analysis (82).

Niacin

The nomenclature of the IUNS is recommended. Measurement of the total niacin content of a food requires preliminary treatment of the sample with acid either on a steam bath or in an autoclave (18).

Colorimetric measurement following reaction with cyanogen bromide (2) or microbiological assay are the suggested methods. *L. arabinosus* ≡ *L. plantarum* (ATCC 8014, NCIB 6376) is probably the most suitable organism, being specific and responding to both nicotinic acid and nicotinamide (2, 7, 18).

Niacin is known to exist in a bound form in many cereals (26, 30) which is unavailable to man as a source of the vitamin. As yet there are no accepted methods for the measurement of available niacin, although the bound forms can be separated by gel-filtration.

Mode of Expression

Niacin activity in a food should be expressed in terms of equivalents (30), which include the contribution from tryptophan (60 mg ≡ 1 mg niacin equivalent). The need for the method of calculation of equivalents to be described in the tables, and the basic analytical values to be given in comprehensive tables is again emphasised.

Folic Acid

The term folacin should be used strictly according to the IUNS proposals (31, 42); that is to include folic acid and related compounds exhibiting qualitatively the biological activity of folic acid. The extraction should be made in the presence of ascorbate as an anti-oxidant (91).

In view of the uncertainty with regard to the absorption of the higher conjugates of folic acid it is suggested that National Food Composition Tables should contain values for 'free folate' measured microbiologically without conjugase treatment. *L. casei* (ATCC 7649, NCIB 6375) is the suggested organism (20, 72).

This procedure will underestimate the total folacin activity in the foodstuff and is suggested as an interim measure until the biological activity of the higher conjugates in man has been studied in more detail.

Vitamin B_{12}

Microbiological assay with *L. leichmannii* (ATCC 7830, NCIB 8118) after conversion to the cyano form is the suggested method of measurement (2, 90).

Tocopherols

It is suggested that the values given in National Food Tables should be limited to the form for which the biological activity is reasonably well-defined, in this case α-tocopherol. The most satisfactory procedures at the present time involve chromatographic separation (24, 81, 82) followed by colorimetric measurement (29, 94).

Vitamin B_6

Microbiological assay with *Saccharomyces carlsbergensis* (ATCC 9080) as the test organism is suggested after preliminary treatment of the sample with either acid or enzymatic hydrolysis (3, 4, 41).

Calculation of Energy Value

The various systems of energy conversion factors which have been used to calculate the energy value of foods were reviewed by *Morey* (59) and more recently by *Widdowson* (100). The work of *Atwater et al.* in particular has been extensively reviewed by *Merrill and Watt* (57). The Specific Energy Factors of *Merrill and Watt* (57) depend very largely on the experimental work of *Atwater et al.* and discount the effect of one food on another in a mixed diet.

Recent work shows that the use of the *Atwater* system of factors, modified by using the heat of combustion of monosaccharide sugars for available carbohydrate (expressed as monosaccharides) gives a reasonably accurate prediction of the metabolizable energy in diets of a type eaten in Western Europe (77).

The suggested energy conversion factors for a number of constituents of food are given in table X. Table X also includes values for the more important organic acids found in foods. In most cases these contribute only small amounts of energy to the total daily intake and they are only significant for a few fruits and fruit products. As they can be completely metabolised within the body and are well absorbed, the energy conversion factor suggested is the same as the heat of combustion, although small amounts of these acids are excreted in the urine under normal conditions.

This is also true for alcohol, except when very large amounts are consumed.

Mode of Expression

According to the principles layed down in the Systeme International, energy values should be expressed in terms of the joule. In nutritional work the conversion factor from the calorie to the joule should be the

Table X. Energy value of some constituents of foods

Substance	Heat of combustion kcal/g	Energy conversion factor	
		kcal/g	kJ/g[1]
Protein	5.65	4.00	16.7
Fat	9.35	9.00	37.7
Available carbohydrate (expressed as monosaccharide)	3.75	3.75	15.7
Ethyl alcohol	7.07	7.00	29.3
Acetic acid	3.49	3.49	14.6
Malic acid	2.39	2.39	10.0
Lactic acid	3.62	3.62	15.1
Citric acid	2.47	2.47	10.3
Glycerol	4.31	4.31	18.0

1 The 'rounding-up' of these values to integers is consistent with the precision with which these factors were derived experimentally, and observed individual variation (57, 65, 77).

thermochemical one, that is 4.184 kJ/kcal (65). At the present time it is desirable to include values for both kcal and kJ in Tables of Food Composition until the majority of users are completely familiar with the use of the joule.

In expressing energy values, the use of more than three significant figures gives a spurious impression of accuracy. This may mean that it is necessary to give the energy value of foods as kilo joules (kJ) per 100 g and to summate total daily energy intakes in terms of megajoules (MJ).

Whichever system of calculation is chosen it is important that the system used is clearly described in the tables.

Format and Textual Matter

Tables of Food Composition are reference documents which may be in constant use; their presentation of data should be such that they may be used quickly, efficiently and accurately.

Careful study of the way in which the tables are used, and discussions with the users, should play an important part in deciding on the type of format which should be adopted.

The textual matter should include information on the methods of analysis and the criteria used in selecting the values given in the tables. Where possible, advice should be given on the confidence which should be attached to the values, and comments on the extent of natural variation in composition made where necessary.

The amount and distribution of textual matter within the tables needs to be varied according to the type of table. In the comprehensive tables, the positioning of the textual matter is probably not critical; in the national tables, however, it is essential that important textual comments are read by the user and care must be taken not to leave these points in the main introduction to the tables where they are unlikely to be read more than once.

Many national tables intersperse text and tables and this may provide a more useful form of presentation for the general user (a list of European Tables of Food Composition is given in the Appendix).

Acknowledgements

Members of the Working Party would like to thank the director of the Stiftung 'im Grüene' for the hospitality at Zurich-Feldbach which provided an ideal environment for their work.

Many workers gave their advice in the final stages of preparation and their help is gratefully acknowledged.

I would also like to acknowledge the assistance of Mrs. *Edna Collinson* and Mr. *W.J. Branch* in the literature-searching and discussions with Miss *A.A. Paul,* Dr. *E.M. Widdowson* and Dr. *E. Kodicek* during the preparation of the guide lines.

References

1 *Ansell, G.B. and Hawthorne, J.N.:* Phospholipids: chemistry, metabolism and function (Elsevier, Amsterdam 1964).

2 Association of Official Agricultural Chemists. Official methods of analysis, 11th ed. (AOAC, Washington 1970).

3 Association of Vitamin Chemists. Methods of vitamin assay, 3rd ed. (Interscience Publ. Inc., New York 1966).

4 *Atkin, L.; Schultz, A.S., and Frey, C.N.:* Yeast microbiological methods for determination of vitamins. Pyridoxine. Industr. Engng. Chem. (analyt. ed.) *15:* 141 (1943).

5 *Atkinson, T.; Fowler, V.R.; Garton, G.A., and Lough, A.K.:* A rapid method for the accurate determination of lipid in animal tissues. Analyst *97:* 562 (1972).

6 *Barton-Wright, E.C.:* The microbiological assay of nicotinic acid in cereals and other products. Biochem. J. *38:* 314 (1944).

7 *Barton-Wright, E.C.:* The theory and practice of the microbiological assay of the vitamin-B complex: together with the assay of selected amino acids and potassium. Analyst *70:* 283 (1945).

8 *Bergmeyer, H.V.:* Methods of enzymic analysis (Academic Press, New York 1965).

9 *Bishop, C.T.:* Gas-liquid chromatography of carbohydrate derivatives; in *Wolfram and Tipson* Advances in carbohydrate chemistry, vol. 19, p. 105 (Academic Press, New York 1964).

10 *Booth, V.H.:* Carotene: its determination in biological materials. (Heffer and Sons, Cambridge 1957).

11 *Booth, V.H.:* The extraction of pigments from plant materials. Analyst *84:* 464 (1959).

12 *Booth, V.H.:* Problems in the determination of FDNB-available lysine. J. Sci. Food Agric. *22:* 658 (1971).

13 *Bowen, H.J.M.:* The determination of chlorine, bromine and iodine in biological materials by activation analysis. Biochem. J. *73:* 381 (1959).

14 *Brunius, E.:* Assay of vitamin-A oils. Nature, Lond. *181:* 395 (1958).

15 *Carpenter, K.J.:* The estimation of the available lysine in animal protein foods. Biochem. J. *77:* 604 (1960).

16 *Carr, F.H. and Price, E.A.:* Colour reactions attributed to vitamin A. Biochem. J. *20:* 497 (1926).

17 *Clegg, K.M.:* The application of the anthrone reagent to the estimation of starch in cereals. J. Sci. Food Agric. *7:* 40 (1956).

18 *Clegg, K.M.; Kodicek, E., and Mistry, S.P.:* A modified medium for *Lactobacillus casei* for the assay of B vitamins. Biochem. J. *50:* 326 (1952).

19 *Cocks, L.V. and Rede, C. van:* Laboratory handbook for oil and fat analysts (Academic Press, New York 1966).

20 *Cooperman, J.M.:* Microbiological assay of serum and whole blood folic acid activity. Amer. J. clin. Nutr. *20:* 1015 (1967).

21 *Coppock, J.B.M.; Knight, R.A., and Vaughan, M.C.:* The moisture content of white bread. Nutrition, Lond. *12:* 63 (1958).

22 *Cotlove, E.; Trantham, H.V., and Bowman, R.L.:* An instrument and method, rapid, accurate and sensitive for the titration of chloride in biologic samples. J. Lab. clin. Med. *51:* 461 (1958).

23 *Dawson, R.M.C.; Elliot, D.C.; Elliot, W.H., and Jones, K.M.:* Data for biochemical research, 2nd ed. (Oxford University Press, London 1969).

24 *Dean, A.C.:* The separation of dimeric tocopherols products from vitamin E in food by dry column chromatography. Chem. Ind. 677 (1971).

25 *Dellweg, H. und Bernhauer, K.:* Über die mikrobiologische Bestimmung von Thiamin mit Hilfe von *Lactobacillus fermenti.* Biochem. Z. *328:* 264 (1956).

26 Department of Health and Social Security. Recommended intakes of nutrients for the United Kingdom. Reports on Publ. Hlth and Med. Subjects, No. 120 (HMSO, London 1969).

27 *Deutsch, M.J. and Weeks, C.E.:* Micro-fluorometric assay for vitamin C. J. Ass. off. Agric. Chem. *48:* 1248 (1965).

28 *Eckschlager, K.:* Errors, measurement and results in chemical analysis (Van Nostrand & Reinhold, London 1969).

29 *Emmerie, A. and Engel, C.:* Colorimetric determination of α-tocopherol (vitamin E) Rec. Trans. Chim. Pays Bas *57:* 1351 (1938).

30 FAO/WHO Expert Group. Requirements of vitamin A. Thiamine, riboflavine and niacin. WHO Techn. Rep. Ser. No. 362 (1967).

31 FAO/WHO Expert Group. Requirements of ascorbic acid, vitamin D, vitamin B_{12} folate and iron. WHO Techn. Rep. Ser. No. 452 (1970).

32 *Fiske, C.H. and Subbarow, Y.:* The colorimetric determination of phosphorus, J. biol. Chem. *66:* 375 (1925).

33 *Fleck, A. and Munro, H.N.:* The determination of organic nitrogen in biological materials. A review. Clin. chim. Acta *11:* 2 (1965).

34 *Floridi, A.:* An improved method for the automated analysis of sugars by ion-exchange chromatography. J. Chromatog. *59:* 61 (1971).

35 *Folch, J.; Lees, M., and Stanley, G.H.S.:* A simple method for the isolation and purification of total lipids from animal tissues. J. biol. Chem. *226:* 497 (1957).

36 *Friedmann, T.E.; Witt, N.F.; Neighbors, B.W., and Weber, C.W.:* Determination of available carbohydrates in plant and animal foods. J. Nutr. *91:* suppl. 2, 10 (1967).

37 *Gehrke, C.W. and Leimer, K.:* Trimethylsilylation of amino acids. Derivatisation and Chromatography. J. Chromatog. *57:* 219 (1971).

38 *Gruen, L.C. and Rivett, D.E.:* Specificity of Spies and Chambers' reagent for colorimetric estimation of tryptophan. Analyt. Biochem. *44:* 519 (1971).

39 *Hallab, A.H. and Epps, E.A.:* Variables affecting the determination of crude fibre. J. Ass. off. Agric. Chem. *46:* 1006 (1963).

40 Hoffmann-La Roche. Methods of vitamin assay – a bibliography (Hoffmann-La Roche, Basle 1959).

41 *Hopkins, R.H. and Pennington, R.J.:* The assay of the vitamin B_6 complex. Biochem. J. *41:* 110 (1947).

42 IUNS Committee on Nomenclature. Tentative rules for generic description and trivial names for vitamins and related compounds. Nutr. Abs. Rev. *40:* 395 (1970).

43 IUPAC. The assay of vitamin A in oils (Butterworths Scientific Publications, London 1959).

44 *Jansen, B.C.P.:* Quantitative Bestimmung von Aneurin (= Vitamin B_1). Z. Vitamin-, Hormon-, Fermentforsch. *7:* 239 (1938).

45 *Jones, D.B.:* Factors for converting percentages of nitrogen in foods and feeds into percentages of protein. US Dept. Agr. Cir. *183:* (1941).

46 *Jonsson, P. and Samuelson, O.:* Automated chromatography of sugars on cation exchange resins. Analyt. Chem. *39:* 1156 (1967).

47 *Kiesler, R.B.:* Rapid quantitative anion exchange chromatography of carbohydrates. Analyt. Chem. *39:* 1416 (1967).

48 *Kodicek, E. and Lawson, D.E.M.:* Vitamin D; in *Gyorgy and Pearson* The vitamins, 2nd ed., vol. VI (Academic Press, New York 1967).

49 *Kodicek, E. and Wang, Y.L.:* The fluorimetric estimation of riboflavin in foodstuffs and other biological material. Biochem. J. *44:* 340 (1949).

50 *Landy, M. and Dicken, D.M.:* A microbiological assay method for six B vitamins using *Lactobacillus casei* and a medium of essentially known composition. J. Lab. clin. Med. *27:* 1086 (1942).

51 *Lindner, K. and Dworschak, E.:* Für Serienuntersuchungen geeignete flammenfotometrische Methode zur Bestimmung von Kalium, Natrium, Calcium und Magnesium in Lebensmitteln. Z. Lebensmitt.Unters. *131:* 207 (1966).

52 *McCance, R.A. and Lawrence, R.D.:* The carbohydrate content of foods. Spec. Rep. Ser. Med. Res. Counc. Lond. No. 135 (HMSO, London 1929).

53 *McCance, R.A.; Widdowson, E.M., and Shackleton, L.R.B.:* The nutritive value of fruits, vegetables and nuts. Spec. Rep. Ser. Med. Res. Counc. Lond. No. 213 (HMSO, London 1936).

54 *Macrae, J.C. and Armstrong, D.G.:* Enzyme method for the determination of α-linked glucose polymers in biological materials. J. Sci. Food Agric. *19:* 578 (1968).

55 *Mangold, D.E.:* The digestion and utilization of crude fibre. Nutr. Abs. Rev. *3:* 647 (1934).

56 *Mergregian, S.:* Rapid spectrophotometric determination of fluoride with zirconium-eriochrome cyanine R. Lake. Analyt. Chem. *26:* 1161 (1954).

57 *Merrill, A.L. and Watt, B.K.:* The energy value of foods – basis and derivation. (US Dept. Agric. Handbook, 74, 1955).

58 *Moore, S.:* On the determination of cystine as cysteic acid. J. biol. Chem. *238:* 235 (1963).

59 *Morey, N.B.:* An analysis and comparison of different methods of calculation of the energy value of diets. Nutr. Abs. Rev. *6:* 1 (1936).

60 *Munro, H.N. and Fleck, A.:* Recent developments in the measurement of nucleic acids in biological materials. Analyst *91:* 78 (1966).

61 *Murray, T.K.; Day, K.C., and Kodicek, E.:* The differentiation and assay of vitamins D_2 and D_3 by gas-liquid chromatography. Biochem. J. *98:* 293 (1966).
62 *Neuman, R.E. and Logan, M.A.:* The determination of hydroxyproline. J. biol. Chem. *184:* 299 (1950).
63 *Porter, J.W.G.; Westgarth, D.R., and Williams, A.P.:* A collaborative test of ion-exchange chromatographic methods for determining amino acids. Brit. J. Nutr. *22:* 437 (1968).
64 *Reid, P.E.; Donaldson, B.; Secret, D.W., and Bradford, B.:* A simple, rapid, isothermal gas chromatographic procedure for the analysis of monosaccharide mixtures. J. Chromatog. *47:* 199 (1970).
65 Report of the Subcommittee on Metrication of the British National Committee for Nutritional Sciences. Metric units, conversion factors and nomenclature in nutritional and food sciences (The Royal Society, London 1972).
66 *Roe, I.H. and Kuetner, C.A.:* The determination of ascorbic acid in whole blood and urine through the 2,4-dinitrophenyl-hydrazine derivative of dehydroascorbic acid. J. biol. Chem. *147:* 399 (1943).
67 *Sandell, E.B.:* Colorimetric determination of traces of metals, 3rd ed. (Interscience Publishers, New York 1959).
68 *Schlenk, H. and Gellerman, J.L.:* Esterification of fatty acids with diazomethane on a small scale. Analyt. Chem. *32:* 1412 (1960).
69 *Schram, E.; Dustin, J.P.; Moore, S. et Bigwood, E.J.:* Application de la chromatographie sur échanges d'ions à l'étude de la composition des aliments en acides aminés. Analyt. chim. Acta *9:* 149 (1953).
70 *Singer, L. and Armstrong, W.D.:* Determination of fluoride in blood serum. Analyt. Chem. *31:* 105 (1959).
71 *Siriwardene, J.A. de S.; Evans, R.A.; Thomas, A.J., and Axford, R.F.E.:* Use of an automated *Kjeldahl* analyser for determination of nitrogen in biological materials; in *Skeggs, Jr.* Automation in analytical chem., p. 144 (Mediad, New York 1966).
72 *Snell, E.E.:* Use of microorganisms for assay of vitamins. Physiol. Rev. *28:* 255 (1948).
73 *Sobel, A.E. and Webbin, H.:* Activated glycerol dichlorohydrin. A new colorimetric reagent for vitamin A. Industr. Engng. Chem. (analyt. ed.) *18:* 570 (1946).
74 *Southgate, D.A.T.:* The determination of carbohydrates in foods. I. Available carbohydrate. J. Sci. Food Agric. *20:* 326 (1969 a).
75 *Southgate, D.A.T.:* The determination of carbohydrates in foods. II. Unavailable carbohydrates. J. Sci. Food Agric. *20:* 331 (1969 b).
76 *Southgate, D.A.T.:* A procedure for the measurement of fats in foods. J. Sci. Food Agric. *22:* 590 (1971).
77 *Southgate, D.A.T. and Durnin, J.V.G.A.:* Calorie conversion factors. An experimental reassessment of the factors used in the calculations of the energy value of human diets. Brit. J. Nutr. *24:* 517 (1970).

78 *Spackman, D.G.; Stein, W.H., and Moore, S.:* Automatic recording apparatus for use in the chromatography of amino acids. Analyt. Chem. *30:* 1190 (1958).

79 *Sperry, W.M.:* Methods of biochemical analysis, vol. 2, p. 83 (Interscience, New York 1955).

80 *Spies, J.R. and Chambers, J.R.:* Chemical determination of tryptophan. Analyt. Chem. *20:* 30 (1948).

81 *Stahl, E.:* Thin layer chromatography. A laboratory handbook (Springer, Berlin; Academic Press, New York 1965).

82 *Stein, M.* (ed.): Proceedings of The University of Nottingham Residential Seminar on Vitamins. *Christie,* p. 146; *Bell,* p. 165 (Churchill, Livingstone; Edinburgh and London, 1971).

83 *Stoffel, W.; Chu, F., and Ahrous, E.H., Jr.:* Analysis of long-chain fatty acids by gas-liquid chromatography. Micromethod for preparation of methyl esters. Analyt. Chem. *31:* 307 (1959)

84 *Stekelenburg, G.J. and Desplanque, J.:* Deproteination by ultrafiltration with centrifugal force. Techniques in amino-acid analysis (Technicon Instruments Co. Ltd., Chertsey 1966).

85 *Strohecker, R. and Henning, M.M.:* Vitamin assay: tested methods (Chemie GmbH, Weinheim 1966).

86 *Sweeley, C.C.; Bentley, R.; Makita, M., and Wells, W.W.:* Gas-liquid chromatography of trimethylsilyl derivatives of sugars and related substances. J. amer. chem. Soc. *85:* 2497 (1963).

87 *Sweeney, J.P. and Marsh, A.C.:* Separation of carotene stereoisomers in vegetables. J. Ass. off. Anal. Chem. *53:* 937 (1970).

88 *Szöke, K.; Kramer, M., and Lindner, K.:* An appropriate method for the rapid esterification of lipids and lipid fractions in series investigators. Fette, Seifen, Anstrichmittel *67:* 257 (1965).

89 The Vitamin B_1 Sub-Committee of the Accessory Food Factors Committee of the Medical Research Council and the Lister Institute. The vitamin B_1 content of national flour and bread – the results of comparative tests by various methods. Biochem. J. *37:* 433 (1943).

90 *Thompson, H.J.; Dietrich, L.S., and Elvehjem, C.A.:* The use of *Lactobacillus leichmannii* in the estimation of vitamin B_{12} activity. J. biol. Chem. *184:* 175 (1950).

91 *Toennies, G.; Uspin, E., and Phillips, P.M.:* Precursors of the folic acid-active factors of blood. J. biol. Chem. *221:* 855 (1956).

92 *Trautner, K.:* Enzymatische Zuckerbestimmungen. Z. Ernährungsw. *8:* (suppl.) 40 (1969).

93 *Tristam, G.R.:* Report of 2nd amino-acid colloquium, 33 (Technicon Instruments Co. Ltd., Chertsey 1964).

94 *Tsen, C.C.:* An improved spectrophotometric method for the determination of tocopherols using 4,7-diphenyl 1,10-phenanthroline. Analyt. Chem. *33:* 884 (1961).

95 *Van Soest, P.J.:* Use of detergents in the analysis of fibrous feeds: (a) preparation of fiber residues of low nitrogen content; (b) a rapid method for the determination of fiber and lignin. J. Ass. off. Agric. Chem. *46:* 825 a, 829 b (1963).
96 *Van Soest, P.J. and Wine, R.H.:* Method for determination of lignin, cellulose and silica. J. anim. Sci. *26:* 940 (1967).
97 *Vastagh, G.:* Die Bestimmung von Vitamin A, besonders in Arzneipräparaten. I. Teil. Arch. Pharm., Weinheim *279:* 51 (1941).
98 *Vuilleumier, J.:* Analytische Probleme bei der Bestimmung von Vitaminen im Zusammenhang mit Ernährungserhebungen. Z. Vitamin-, Hormon-, Fermentforsch. *37:* 504 (1967).
99 *Watt, B.K. and Merrill, A.L.:* Composition of foods (US Dept. Agric. Handbook, No. 8, 1963).
100 *Widdowson, E.M.:* Assessment of the energy value of human foods. Proc. Nutr. Soc. *14:* 142 (1955).
101 *Wilson, P.W.; Lawson, D.E.M., and Kodicek, E.:* Gas-liquid chromatography of ergocalciferol and cholecalciferol in nanogram quantities. J. Chromatog. *39:* 75 (1969).

Appendix

European Food Composition Tables

(Based on the FAO Annotated Bibliography on Food Composition Tables, FAO, Rome, 1969)

Belgium. A selection of tables covering the foods from different regions prepared by the Centre de Recherches Zootechniques de Lovenjoul (Louvain). Director Prof. *A. De Vuyst.*

Denmark. Rich Ege-Nyt: Føderare-og ernae ringstabeller (Nordish Forlag, Arnold Busck, Copenhagen 1969).

Finland. O. Turpeinen and P. Roine: Ruoka-Aine-Taulukko, 5th ed. (1967).

France. L. Randoin, P. Le Gallic, Y. Dupuis et A. Beradin: Tables de composition des aliments, 3rd ed. (Institut Scientifique d'Hygiène Alimentaire, Centre National de la Recherche Scientifique, *J. Janore* (ed.) (Paris, 1961).

Germany. S.W. Souci, W. Fauchmann und H. Kraut: Die Zusammensetzung der Lebensmittel, Nährwert-Tabellen (Wissenschaftliche Verlagsgesellschaft mbH, Stuttgart 1962, 1964).

Greece. S.A. Kaloyereas: Chemical composition of Greek foods (Ministry of Agriculture, Athens 1952).

Hungary. R. Tarjan and K. Lindner: Food composition tables, 7th ed. (Budapest 1972).

Italy. Composizione in alcuni principi nutritivi e valore calorico degli alimenti comunemente consumati in Italia (National Institute of Nutrition, Rome 1968).

Netherlands. C. Den Hartog (ed.): Nederlandse voedingsmiddelen tabel, 26th ed. (Uitgave het Voorlichtingsbureau voor de Voeding 1971).

Norway. Naerings middel tabell, 3rd ed. (Landsforeningen for Kosthold of Helse, Oslo 1966).

Poland. A. Szczygka (ed.): Tabele skladu 1 wartosci odzywczych produktow spozywczych (Panstwowy Zaktad Wydawnictw Lekarskich, Warsaw 1972).

Portugal. F.A. Goncalves Ferreira and M.E. Da Silva Crasa: Tabela de composicao dos alimentos (Ministry of Health and Assistance, Lisbon 1961).

Spain. Tablas de composicion de alimentos (University of Madrid, School of Bromatology).

Sweden. E. Abramson: Kost tabell (Svenskca Bokförlaget Bonniers, Stockholm 1971).

Switzerland. O. Högl und E. Lauber: Nährwert der Lebensmittel (reprinted from Schweizerisches Lebensmittelbuch, Bern 1961).

United Kingdom. R.A. McCance and E.M. Widdowson: The composition of foods (Medical Research Council Special Report No. 297, HMSO London 1960, reprinted 1967 and 1969).

USSR. T.E. Boldyrev and O.P. Molcanova (eds.): Tables of chemical composition and nutritive value of food products (Medgiz, Moscow 1954).

Yugoslavia. R. Buzina (ed.): Tablice sastava zivotrih namirnica (Dubrovnik 1972).

The list is confined to the more recent series of tables. Most of the tables would fall within the definition of 'National' used in the 'guide lines', with the exception of the German one which is more comprehensive.

Author's address: Dr. *D.A.T. Southgate,* Dunn Nutritional Laboratory, University of Cambridge and Medical Research Council, *Cambridge* (England)

A Brief History of British Food Composition Tables

Elsie M. Widdowson

Dunn Nutritional Laboratory, University of Cambridge and Medical Research Council, Cambridge

It was the shortages of food in the First World War that led to the first British food composition tables. Before that time, extensive tables had already been published in America and in Germany. *Atwater* began his investigations of food for man and animals in 1869, while he was still a student at the Sheffield Scientific School of Yale University. He continued this work for many years and it culminated with the publication in 1896 of USDA Bulletin No. 28 'The Chemical Composition of American Food Materials'. Some of the values given in the original publication still appear in the current tables of food composition used in the United States (USDA Agricultural Handbook No. 8). The first European tables were prepared by *König* in 1908, and an 18th edition of *Schall*'s tables, based largely on these early values, is still widely used in Germany.

During the First World War, the War Office in Britain directed Captain *Plimmer,* a chemist serving in the Army, to make analyses of all common British foods. This was expecting rather a lot of one young man, but *Plimmer,* in the tradition of the Army, obeyed, though with some misgivings. He says in his introduction to the tables 'Such a complete set of data as those of *Atwater and Bryant* could not be obtained by a single worker in the limited period of time available, but in the time so devoted, analyses of most foodstuffs have been made: analyses number about 900. It is perhaps of interest that the number of weighings involved were over 20,000. Each analysis, in so far as material was available, was carried out in duplicate, and the mean figure is given. This part of the work was carried out single-handed.' It is perhaps salutary to consider that one man made determinations of water, ash, protein, carbohydrate and fat in 900 foods, and fibre and chloride as well in many of them. The tables entitled 'Analyses and Energy Values of Foods' were published in 1921.

That year was important in the history of British tables of food composition in another respect. Insulin was discovered, just in time to save the life of Dr. *R.D. Lawrence* of King's College Hospital, London, who had severe diabetes. Dr. *Lawrence* had gone to Italy to practise medicine for as long as he could, and probably to end his days there. He returned to King's and devoted his whole working life to the treatment of persons with diabetes. *R.A. McCance* was a medical student at King's at that time, and he had been given a small grant for work in his spare moments, in the then newly created biochemical department. He, too, became interested in the treatment of diabetes.

Fruit and vegetables were then the mainstay of diabetic diets, but there were two difficulties about calculating their food value. First, the figures for protein and fat given by different authors were uniform enough, but the values for carbohydrate, nearly all determined 'by difference', might vary by several hundred per cent: carbohydrate in parsnips, for example, might be 21 % or 2 %, according to which table one chose to use. Second, almost all previous analyses had been carried out on raw materials, but people eat cooked foods, and *Lawrence* knew that the carbohydrate content of many foods must be altered by cooking.

In 1925, the British Medical Research Council gave *McCance* a grant to enable him to analyse cooked and raw fruits and vegetables for available carbohydrate, and he began to try to separate the available readily soluble sugars and starch from the relatively unavailable pentosans, hemicelluloses, and cellulose. He, like *Plimmer,* did this analytical work single-handed, along with his medical duties; he dealt with 109 different plant materials, each on six separate occasions. He hydrolyzed the fruit or vegetable with hydrochloric acid, then neutralised, and determined the total reducing sugars. The results of this work were published in 1929 as a Medical Research Council Special Report by *McCance and Lawrence,* 'The Carbohydrate Content of Foods'. The value of this report, lies not so much in the figures it gives for carbohydrate in fruit and vegetables, but in its second and by far longest part, a thoughtful review which Dr. *McCance* wrote, of the food value of vegetable carbohydrates. This is a classic, and is as true today as when it was written.

Before this report was published, the manuscript was submitted to Prof. *E.P. Cathcart* of Glasgow University. Prof. *Cathcart* was interested in the whole subject of nutrition and he at once said that, from the point of view of general nutrition, protein and fat were more important than carbohydrate; he thought it was a great pity that these constituents had not been determined as well as carbohydrate. Dr. *McCance* told Prof. *Cathcart* that he was willing to analyse foods for protein and fat, and also for minerals, if he could be provided with some assistance, but he really could not go on doing this work, as well as being a doctor, all alone. The results of this was that *H.L. Shipp* joined Dr. *McCance* at King's College Hospital in 1930, and a detailed study of the composition of meat and fish began.

Continuing with the idea that it was important to know the composition of cooked food, Dr. *McCance* and Mr. *Shipp* included in their work an investigation of the losses of various constituents from meat and fish when cooked in various ways. The results of this study were published in 1933 under the title of 'The Chemistry of Flesh Foods and Their Losses on Cooking'.

Mr. *H.L. Shipp* left Dr. *McCance* in 1933 and was replaced by *L.R.B. Shackleton,* the plan being that fruits and vegetables should now be analysed for protein, fat, and minerals, their available carbohydrate content having already been measured.

It was in 1933, just as this new study on fruit and vegetables was beginning, that I first met Dr. *McCance.* It so happened, that I knew something about the determination of carbohydrate in fruit, for I had recently finished a doctoral thesis on the carbohydrate content of developing apples. I told Dr. *McCance* that his previous values for carbohydrate in fruit were undoubtedly all too low, for much of the carbohydrate in fruit is present as fructose, and this would have been partially destroyed by boiling with acid. Instead of being annoyed, as he well might have been, he at once asked me whether I would join him and *Shackleton* in the new analyses of fruits and vegetables which were just beginning, and repeat the determination of carbohydrate by more accurate methods.

We eventually analysed all common fruits, vegetables and nuts for water, nitrogen, fat (where present), minerals and the separate 'available' carbohydrate fractions, starch and dextrin, sucrose, glucose and fructose. Vegetables that are generally eaten cooked were analysed after cooking, and we again studied the losses of soluble constituents on cooking. The results were published in 1936 under the title 'The Nutritive Value of Fruits, Vegetables and Nuts'. The stocks of these first three publications were all destroyed in a fire started by enemy action during World War II, and they have been out of print ever since.

My contacts with dietitians and my own individual dietary surveys in the thirties made me realise how much we needed comprehensive tables of the composition of British foods. Meat, fish, fruit and vegetables had now been extensively analysed, so that there now remained cereal foods, dairy products, and items such as beverages, preserves and sweets. If these were also analysed we should have all the material we needed for making a practical set of food tables. We decided to do this, and we embarked on an analysis of these other foods, and that is how the first edition of 'The Chemical Composition of Foods' came to be conceived and born. The tables evolved through a series of happy coincidences, all dating back to the discovery of insulin by *Banting and Best.* The tables were not published until 1940, after we had moved to Cambridge, although most of the work represented in them had been done in London.

In making these tables we departed from food table tradition in several ways. First, the composition of cooked foods was often given, and a section was included on the composition of cooked dishes containing several ingredients. The dishes were prepared and cooked according to recipes, the losses in weight at all stages were measured, and the composition of the final dish calculated from the known composition of all the ingredients. Second, in order to obtain representative figures for the composition of foods, it is clearly necessary to analyse more than one sample. Earlier, workers had generally analysed several samples separately and then calculated the average representative figure. We reduced the amount of work involved by collecting together a number of different samples of each food and mixing them together before we started the analysis. Thus, we obtained no information about the variation in composition between different samples, but it was the representative figure that was generally wanted, and, even after cutting the work down in this way, the tables represented about 10,000 separate determinations, each one made in duplicate.

The shortage of some foods during World War II and afterwards, and the introduction of foods which had not been much used in times of plenty, made it desirable to revise the food tables, and a second edition was published in 1946. The original analytical figures were not altered except in a few instances, but the values for calories were all recalculated since there had been a mistake in the original method of calculation. The tables were extended to include the composition of economically cooked dishes, such as were commonly being prepared at that time, besides the composition of such foods as 85 percent extraction national flour and the bread made from it, which we were using in England in wartime, and dried skim milk, and dried eggs.

Another set of food tables was published in Britain in 1945 'Nutritive Values of Wartime Foods'. These were compiled by the Accessory Food Factors Committee of the Medical Research Council. The figures for many of the foods were taken from our 'Chemical Composition of Foods', but other foods were included, and the emphasis was on raw, rather than cooked, foods. Values for calcium, iron, vitamin A potency, thiamine, and ascorbic acid were included. These tables are now out of print.

In the early 1950s, the time seemed to be ripe for us to begin the preparation of a third edition of our tables. The first two had no figures for vitamins, for methods in those days had not seemed precise enough to warrant any attempt to include them. Techniques had improved, however, and we decided to include them in the third edition. We had Dr. *W.I.M. Holman* with us at that time, and he undertook the responsibility of reading and abstracting every paper on the vitamin content of food published during the past 15–20 years that he could find. This involved studying well over 1,000 papers. There was so much information, particularly about certain foods, such as milk, that we decided it was foolish for us to try to analyse every food for every vitamin, and we agreed to depart from our own policy and to use published values for the vitamins in foods.

With Dr. *Holman*'s special knowledge about methods of vitamin assay, he was able to select the papers which reported results likely to be reliable. He wrote summaries of all these papers, and his opinion of them, on punched cards. He got this far, and then left us to go to South Africa. We were fortunate in finding Miss *I.M. Barrett* when Dr. *Holman* left. She took over all of his records and spent about a year going through these abstracts, recording the values once again on other cards, which were indexed under 'foods'. Finally, she and I went through all of her summaries together, and between us, decided on the figure for each food which we thought most nearly represented the amount of the vitamin in that food.

Another way in which we extended the tables was by including figures for amino acids. Again, the tables are largely a compilation of other workers' values, though some of the figures are our own.

With the help of Dr. *D.A.T. Southgate,* who joined us in 1955, we added about 100 new foods, which we analysed for protein, fat, carbohydrate and minerals, just as we had done before. Many were proprietary preparations which had come on the market since the second edition, or become much more popular after the war. The third edition of our tables, now called 'The Composition of Foods' was published in 1960. This still contained almost all of the values given in the first edition, as well as additional values for new foods and other nutrients.

In 1969, it was decided to begin the preparation of a fourth edition, which would involve a critical appraisal of all the old values, and a considerable amount of analytical work. This work is now under way. It is a collaborative venture of the Medical Research Council, the Ministry of Agriculture, Fisheries and Food, and the Laboratory of the Government Chemist under the overall direction of Dr. *D.A.T. Southgate,* and it is hoped that the new tables will appear in 1975.

Author's address: Dr. *Elsie M. Widdowson,* Department of Investigative Medicine, University of Cambridge, *Cambridge* (England)